POCKET ATLAS OF
MRI MUSCULOSKELETAL ANATOMY

Pocket Atlas of MRI Musculoskeletal Anatomy

Thomas H. Berquist, M.D., F.A.C.R.
Professor of Radiology
Mayo Medical School
Chair, Department of Diagnostic Radiology
Mayo Clinic Jacksonville
Jacksonville, Florida

LIPPINCOTT WILLIAMS & WILKINS
A **Wolters Kluwer** Company
Philadelphia · Baltimore · New York · London
Buenos Aires · Hong Kong · Sydney · Tokyo

Made in the United States of America

Library of Congress Cataloging-in-Publication Data

Berquist, Thomas H. (Thomas Henry), 1945–
    Pocket atlas of MRI musculoskeletal anatomy / Thomas H. Berquist.   p.   cm.
      ISBN 0-7817-0337-9
      1. Musculoskeletal system—Magnetic resonance imaging—Atlases. I. Title.
      [DNLM: 1. Musculoskeletal System—anatomy & histology—atlases. 2. Musculoskeletal System—anatomy & histology—handbooks. 3. Magnetic Resonance Imaging—atlases. 4. Magnetic Resonance Imaging—handbooks. WE 17 B532p 1995]
    QM100.B47 1995
    611'.7—dc20
    DNLM/DLC
    for Library of Congress   95-16479
                                                    CIP

9 8 7 6 5 4 3

Contents

Preface

This pocket atlas is designed to be a portable reference for anatomy of the musculoskeletal system. The head and spine are not included. Images are displayed in the axial, coronal, and sagittal planes, which are commonly used for magnetic resonance imaging. It is especially important to become familiar with sagittal and coronal anatomy as it applies to routine magnetic resonance practice.

Most images are presented using spin-echo sequences, typically T1-weighted or proton density sequences. Slice thickness varies depending on location. Thinner sections (3 to 5mm) were used in the joints, and 0.5- to 1-cm thick sections in extra-articular regions.

The anatomy is labeled using numbers with legends at the top of each page. An illustration demonstrating the level and plane of section is provided for each anatomic section.

This atlas will be useful to physicians who interpret or request magnetic resonance image studies and to fellows, residents, and medical students for review of musculoskeletal anatomy.

POCKET ATLAS OF
MRI MUSCULOSKELETAL ANATOMY

Shoulder Coil

1, acromion
2, clavicle
3, acromioclavicular joint
4, trapezius muscle

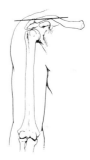

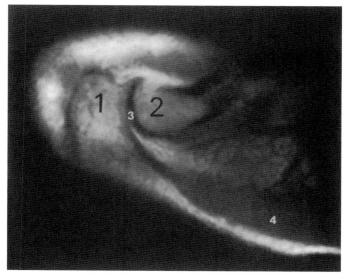

Lateral   SE 500/20   Medial

Shoulder Coil
1, superior humeral head
2, clavicle
3, scapular spine
4, deltoid muscle
5, supraspinatus muscle
6, infraspinatus muscle
7, trapezius muscle

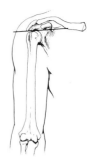

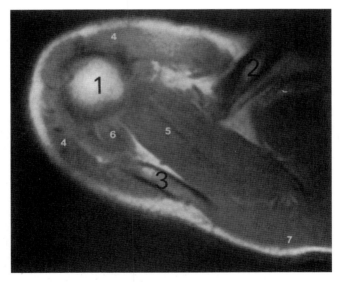

Lateral   SE 500/20   Medial

Shoulder Coil
1, humeral head
2, coracoid
3, scapular spine
4, deltoid muscle
5, infraspinatus muscle
6, supraspinatus muscle
7, subclavius muscle

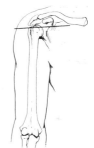

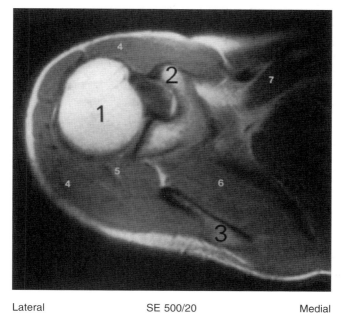

Lateral   SE 500/20   Medial

Shoulder Coil

1, humeral head
2, glenoid
3, biceps tendon
4, deltoid muscle
5, infraspinatus muscle
6, subscapularis muscle
7, coracobrachialis muscle

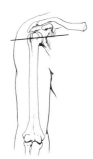

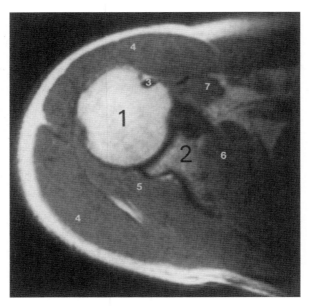

Lateral   SE 500/20   Medial

Shoulder Coil

1, deltoid muscle
2, trapezius muscle
3, clavicle
4, coracoid
5, lesser tuberosity
6, greater tuberosity
7, subscapularis muscle
8, supraspinatus muscle
9, biceps tendon

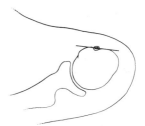

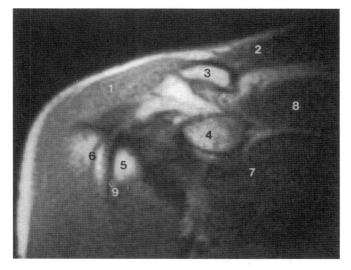

SE 500/20

Shoulder Coil

1, acromion
2, clavicle
3, glenoid
4, deltoid muscle
5, supraspinatus muscle
6, supraspinatus tendon
7, subscapularis muscle
8, coracobrachialis muscle

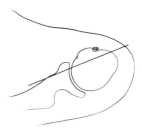

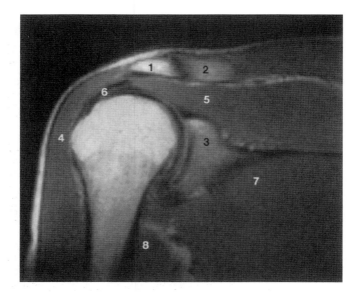

Shoulder Coil
1, acromion
2, glenoid
3, trapezius muscle
4, supraspinatus muscle
5, supraspinatus tendon
6, deltoid muscle
7, humeral head
8, teres major muscle
9, suprascapular artery and
   nerve

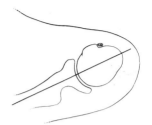

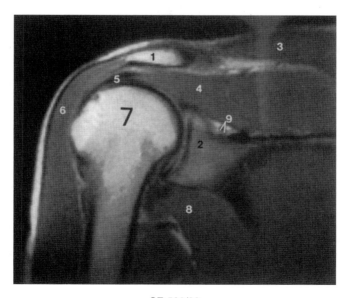

SE 500/20

Shoulder Coil

1, acromion
2, humeral head
3, glenoid
4, trapezius muscle
5, supraspinatus muscle
6, deltoid muscle
7, inferior glenoid labrum

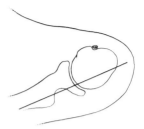

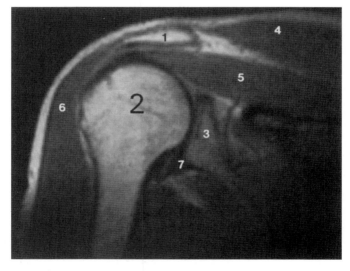

SE 500/20

Shoulder Coil

1, humeral head
2, supraspinatus tendon
3, infraspinatus tendon
4, deltoid muscle
5, teres minor muscle
6, teres major muscle
7, infraspinatus muscle

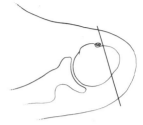

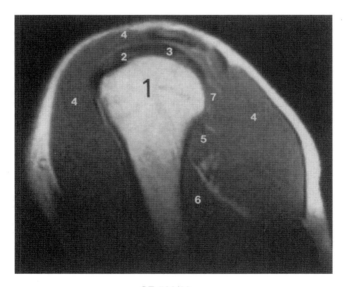

SE 500/20

Shoulder Coil

1, humeral head
2, acromion
3, deltoid muscle
4, supraspinatus muscle and tendon
5, infraspinatus muscle and tendon
6, biceps tendon
7, teres minor muscle
8, pectoralis major muscle

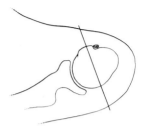

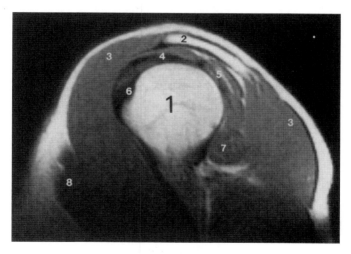

SE 500/20

Shoulder Coil

1, humeral head
2, acromion
3, acromion clavicular joint
4, deltoid muscle
5, supraspinatus muscle and tendon
6, infraspinatus muscle
7, teres minor muscle
8, coracobrachialis muscle

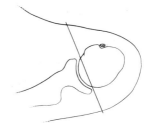

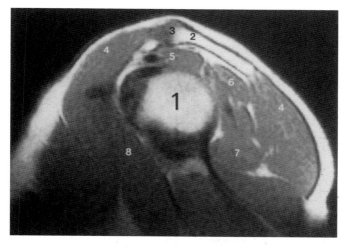

SE 500/20

Shoulder Coil
1, glenoid
2, acromion
3, clavicle
4, coracoid
5, subscapularis muscle
6, coracobrachialis muscle
7, deltoid muscle
8, supraspinatus muscle and tendon
9, infraspinatus muscle
10, teres minor muscle
11, pectoralis major muscle

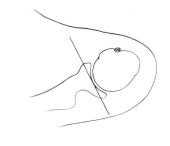

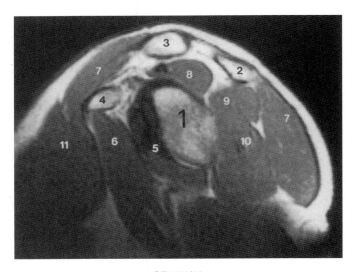

SE 500/20

Shoulder Coil
1, clavicle
2, coracoid
3, scapular spine
4, supraspinatus muscle
5, subscapularis muscle
6, deltoid muscle
7, infraspinatus muscle
8, pectoralis major muscle
9, pectoralis minor muscle

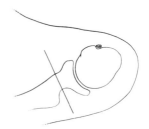

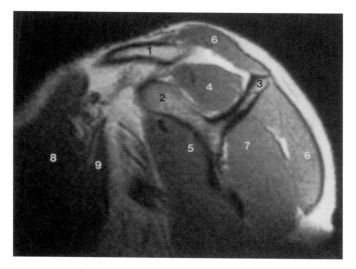

SE 500/20

License Plate Coil
1, humerus
2, deltoid muscle
3, long head of triceps muscle
4, latissimus dorsi and teres
   major muscles
5, short head of biceps muscle
6, biceps tendon, long head
7, pectoralis major muscle
8, axillary artery and vein, and
   brachial plexus

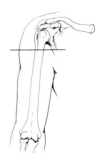

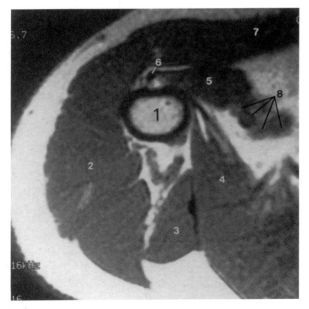

Lateral   SE 500/11   Medial

License Plate Coil

1, humerus
2, deltoid muscle
3, triceps muscle, lateral head
4, triceps muscle, long head
5, triceps muscle, medial head
6, coracobrachialis muscle
7, biceps muscle, long head
8, brachial artery and vein, and
   median and ulnar nerves
9, radial nerve

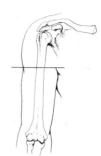

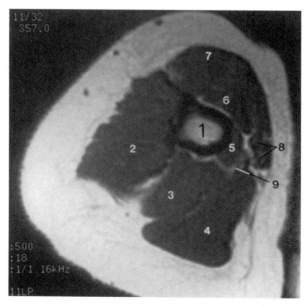

Lateral   SE 500/18   Medial

License Plate Coil

1, humerus
2, long and short heads of biceps muscle
3, coracobrachialis muscle
4, brachial artery, vein, median and ulnar nerves
5, radial nerve
6, triceps muscle, medial head
7, triceps muscle, long head
8, triceps muscle, lateral head

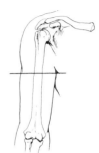

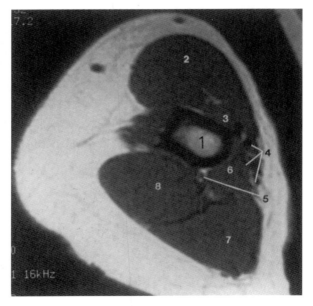

Lateral   SE 500/18   Medial

License Plate Coil

1, humerus
2, biceps muscle, long and
   short heads
3, brachialis muscle
4, basilic vein
5, median nerve
6, ulnar nerve
7, brachial artery
8, triceps muscle, long head
9, triceps muscle, lateral
   head
10, radial nerve
11, cephalic vein

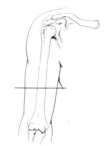

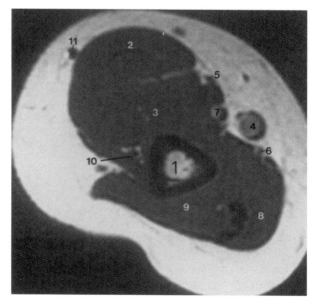

Lateral   SE 500/18   Medial

License Plate Coil
1, humerus
2, biceps muscle
3, brachialis muscle
4, basilic vein
5, median nerve
6, ulnar nerve
7, triceps muscle
8, radial nerve

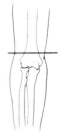

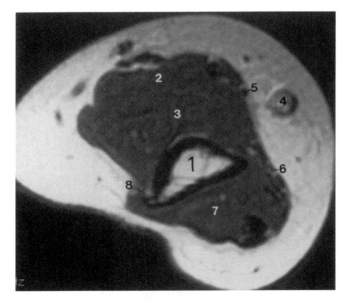

Lateral   SE 500/18   Medial

License Plate Coil
1, humerus
2, deltoid muscle
3, biceps muscle
4, triceps muscle
5, posterior fat pad

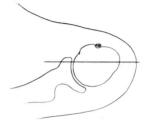

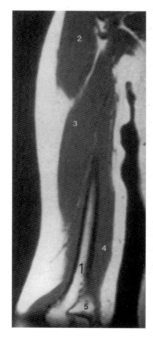

Lateral   SE 500/11   Medial

License Plate Coil
1, humerus
2, deltoid muscle
3, biceps muscle
4, brachialis muscle
5, triceps muscle

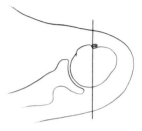

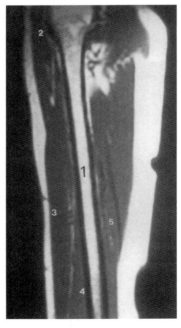

Anterior   SE 500/18   Posterior

Extremity Coil
1, humerus
2, triceps muscle
3, triceps tendon
4, brachialis muscle
5, biceps muscle and tendon
6, brachial artery
7, median nerve
8, ulnar nerve
9, brachioradialis muscle
10, radial nerve

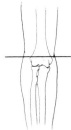

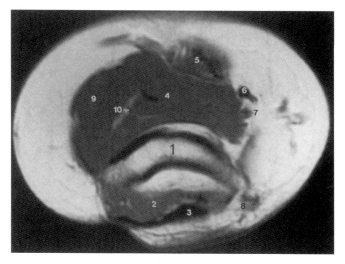

Lateral   SE 500/11   Medial

Extremity Coil
1, olecranon
2, medial epicondyle
3, lateral epicondyle
4, ulnar nerve
5, pronator teres muscle
6, median nerve
7, brachialis muscle
8, brachioradialis muscle
9, radial nerve

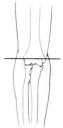

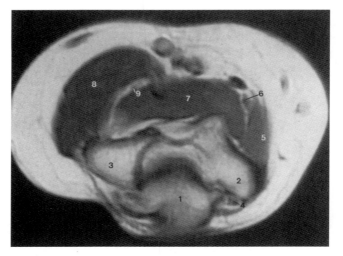

Lateral   SE 500/11   Medial

Extremity Coil
1, radial head
2, ulna
3, anconeus muscle
4, extensor digitorum muscle
5, extensor carpi radialis
   longus muscle
6, brachioradialis muscle
7, brachialis muscle
8, radial nerve
9, biceps tendon
10, flexor digitorum profundus
    muscle
11, pronator teres muscle
12, ulnar nerve

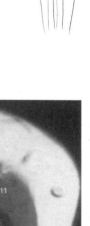

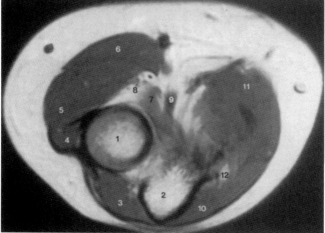

Lateral   SE 500/11   Medial

Extremity Coil

1, radius
2, ulna
3, anconeus muscle
4, extensor carpi ulnaris
   muscle
5, extensor digitorum muscle
6, extensor carpi radialis
   longus muscle
7, deep radial nerve
8, supinator muscle
9, brachioradialis muscle
10, flexor carpi ulnaris muscle
11, flexor digitorum profundus
    muscle
12, ulnar nerve
13, flexor digitorum
    superficialis muscle
14, flexor carpi radialis muscle
15, pronator teres muscle
16, median nerve

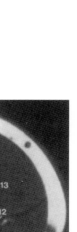

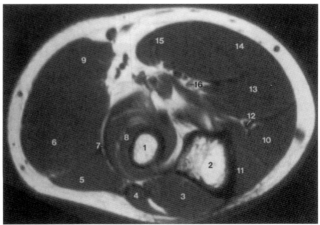

Lateral   SE 500/11   Medial

Extremity Coil

1, radius
2, ulna
3, supinator muscle
4, extensor carpi ulnaris muscle
5, extensor digitorum muscle
6, deep radial nerve
7, extensor carpi radialis muscles
8, brachioradialis muscle
9, superficial radial nerve
10, pronator teres muscle
11, flexor carpi radialis muscle
12, flexor digitorum superficialis muscle
13, ulnar nerve
14, flexor carpi ulnaris muscle
15, flexor digitorum profundus muscle
16, median nerve

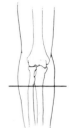

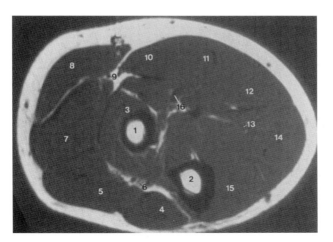

Lateral   SE 500/11   Medial

Extremity Coil
1, trochlea
2, capitellum
3, radial head
4, ulna
5, radial tuberosity
6, brachialis muscle
7, brachioradialis muscle
8, supinator muscle
9, pronator teres muscle
10, flexor carpi radialis muscle
11, extensor carpi radialis
    longus muscle

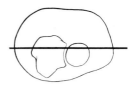

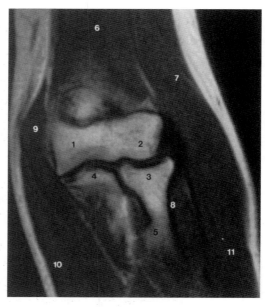

Lateral   SE 500/11   Medial

Extremity Coil
1, medial epicondyle
2, olecranon fossa
3, ulna
4, radial head
5, pronator teres muscle
6, palmaris longus muscle
7, brachioradialis muscle

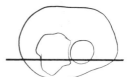

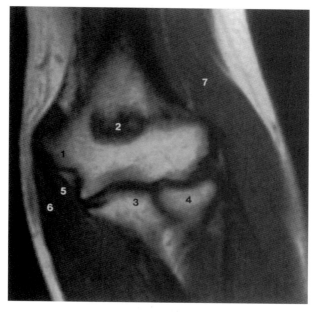

Medial   SE 500/11   Lateral

Extremity Coil

1, triceps tendon
2, triceps muscle
3, trochlea
4, olecranon
5, posterior fat pad
6, brachialis muscle
7, biceps muscle

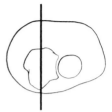

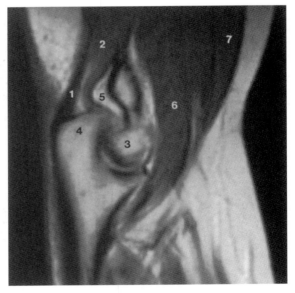

Posterior   SE 500/11   Anterior

Extremity Coil
1, humerus
2, capitellum
3, radial head
4, posterior fat pad
5, triceps muscle
6, brachialis muscle
7, biceps muscle
8, supinator muscle
9, brachioradialis muscle

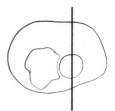

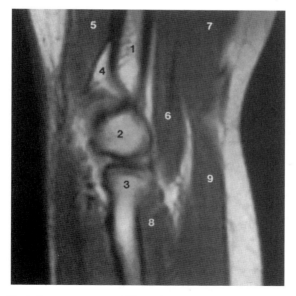

Posterior   SE 500/11   Anterior

Extremity Coil

1, radius
2, ulna
3, pronator teres muscle
4, flexor carpi radialis muscle
5, flexor digitorum
   superficialis muscle
6, ulnar nerve
7, flexor carpi ulnaris muscle
8, flexor digitorum profundus
   muscle
9, extensor carpi ulnaris
   muscle
10, extensor digitorum muscle
11, deep radial nerve
12, supinator muscle
13, median nerve
14, extensor carpi radialis
   muscle
15, brachioradialis muscle

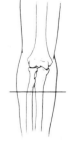

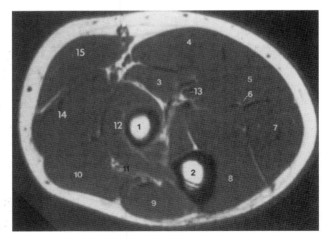

Lateral   SE 500/11   Medial

Extremity Coil
1, radius
2, ulna
3, flexor carpi radialis muscle
4, palmaris longus muscle
5, flexor digitorum
   superficialis muscle
6, ulnar nerve
7, flexor carpi ulnaris muscle
8, flexor digitorum profundus
   muscle
9, interosseous membrane
10, extensor carpi ulnaris
    muscle
11, extensor digiti minimi
    muscle
12, extensor digitorum muscle
13, supinator muscle
14, median nerve
15, brachioradialis

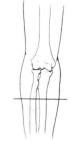

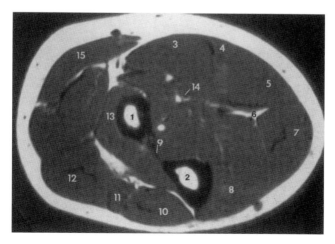

Lateral   SE 500/11   Medial

Extremity Coil
1, radius
2, ulna
3, interosseous membrane
4, extensor carpi ulnaris muscle
5, extensor pollicis muscles
6, flexor digitorum profundus muscle
7, flexor pollicis longus muscle
8, median nerve

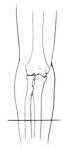

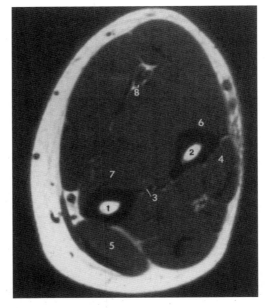

Lateral   SE 500/11   Medial

Extremity Coil

1, radius
2, ulna
3, pronator quadratus muscle
4, flexor carpi ulnaris muscle
5, ulnar nerve
6, flexor digitorum profundus tendons
7, flexor pollicis longus tendon
8, flexor carpi radialis tendon
9, palmaris longus tendon
10, flexor digitorum superficialis tendons
11, extensor carpi ulnaris tendon
12, extensor digitorum and indicis tendons
13, extensor pollicis longus tendon
14, extensor carpi radialis brevis tendon
15, extensor carpi radialis longus tendon

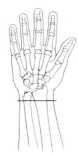

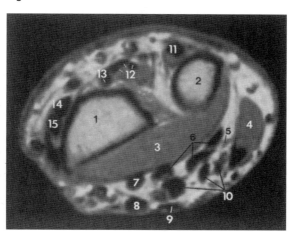

SE 2000/20

Extremity Coil

1, radius
2, ulna
3, dorsal radial tubercle
4, flexor carpi ulnaris muscle
5, ulnar nerve
6, ulnar artery
7, flexor digitorum profundus tendons
8, flexor digitorum superficialis tendons
9, palmaris longus tendon
10, median nerve
11, flexor carpi radialis tendon
12, abductor pollicis longus tendon
13, extensor carpi radialis longus tendon
14, extensor carpi radialis brevis tendon
15, extensor pollicis longus tendon
16, extensor digitorum and indicis tendons
17, extensor carpi ulnaris tendon

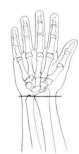

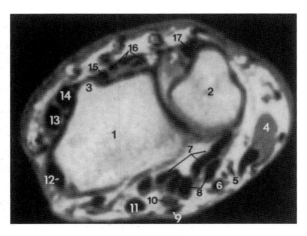

SE 2000/20

Extremity Coil

1, pisiform
2, triquetrum
3, capitate
4, scaphoid
5, ulnar nerve
6, ulnar artery
7, flexor digitorum profundus tendons
8, median nerve
9, palmaris longus tendon
10, flexor carpi radialis tendon
11, flexor pollicis longus tendon
12, extensor carpi ulnaris tendon
13, extensor digitorum and indicis tendon
14, extensor carpi radialis brevis tendon

15, extensor carpi radialis longus and extensor pollicis longus tendons

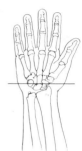

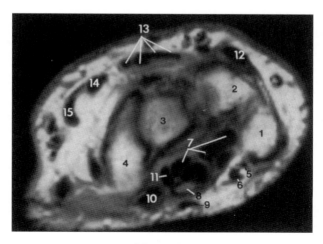

SE 2000/20

Extremity Coil

1, 1st metacarpal base
2, trapezium
3, trapezoid
4, capitate
5, hamate
6, opponeus pollicis muscle
7, abductor digiti minimi muscle
8, ulnar nerve
9, ulnar artery
10, flexor digitorum profundus tendons
11, flexor digitorum superficialis tendons
12, median nerve
13, extensor digiti minimi tendon
14, extensor digitorum and indicis tendons
15, extensor carpi radialis longus tendon

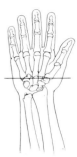

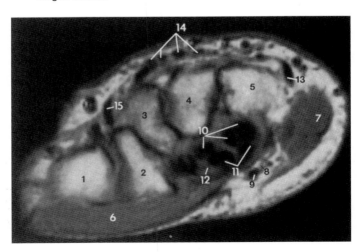

SE 2000/20

Extremity Coil

1, 1st metacarpal head
2–5, 2nd–5th metacarpals
6, abductor digiti minimi muscle
7, opponens digiti minimi muscle
8, palmar aponeurosis
9, flexor digitorum profundus tendons
10, flexor digitorum superficialis tendons
11, abductor pollicis brevis and opponens pollicis muscles
12, flexor pollicis longus tendon
13, abductor pollicis muscle

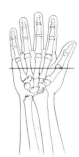

Di, dorsal interosseous muscles
Pi, palmar interosseous muscles

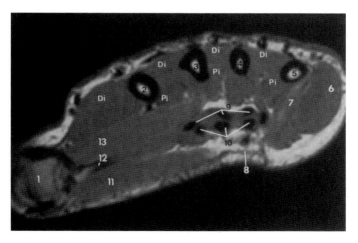

SE 2000/20

Extremity Coil

1, 1st proximal phalanx
2–5, 2nd–5th metacarpals
6, abductor digiti minimi
   muscle
7, opponens digiti minimi
   muscle
8, flexor digitorum
   profundus tendons
9, flexor digitorum
   superficialis tendons
10, abductor pollicis muscle

Di, dorsal interosseous
   muscles
Pi, palmar interosseous
   muscles

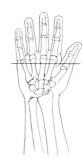

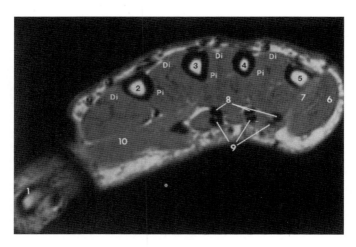

SE 2000/20

Extremity Coil
1, lumbrical muscles
2–5, 2nd–5th metacarpals
6, flexor digitorum
    profundus and
    superficialis tendons
7, abductor digiti minimi
    muscle

Pi, palmar interosseous
    muscles

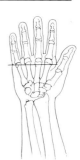

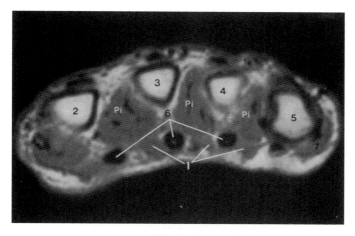

SE 2000/20

Extremity Coil

1, flexor digitorum profundus
   and superficialis tendons
2, 2nd metacarpal
3, 3rd metacarpal
4, 4th metacarpal
5, 5th proximal phalanx
6, extensor tendons

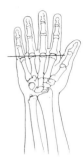

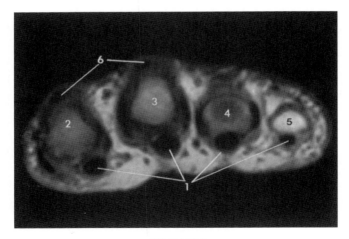

SE 2000/20

Extremity Coil

1, radius
2, ulna
3, trapezoid
4, capitate
5, hamate
6, 2nd metacarpal base
7, 5th metacarpal
8, dorsal capsule 3rd
   metacarpophalangeal joint

Di, dorsal interosseous
    muscles

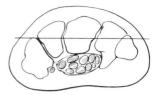

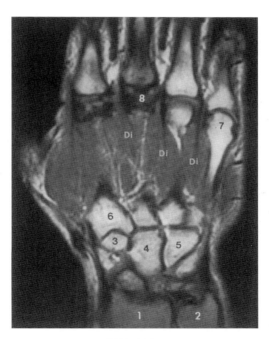

SE 2000/20

Extremity Coil

1, scaphoid
2, lunate
3, triquetrum
4, trapezoid
5, capitate
6, hamate
7, 5th metacarpal
8, adductor pollicis muscle
9, triangular fibrocartilage
10, abductor digiti minimi
muscle

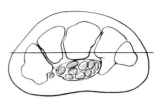

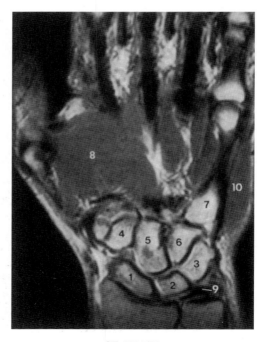

SE 2000/20

Extremity Coil
1, 1st metacarpal
2, trapezium
3, scaphoid
4, flexor tendons
5, hook of hamate
6, flexor pollicis longus tendon
7, abductor digiti minimi
    muscle

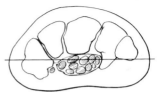

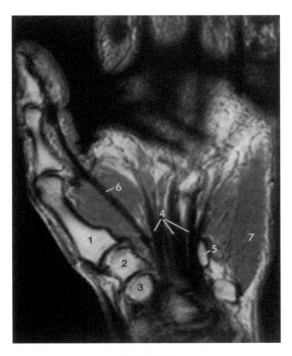

SE 2000/20

Extremity Coil
1, 2nd metacarpal
2, trapezium
3, trapezoid
4, scaphoid
5, adductor pollicis muscle
6, flexor pollicis longus tendon
7, abductor pollicis brevis
   muscle

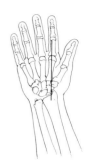

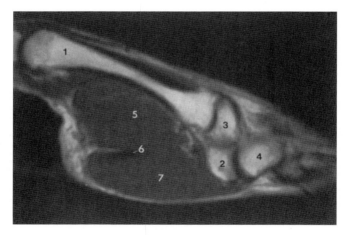

SE 2000/20

Extremity Coil
1, radius
2, lunate
3, capitate
4, 3rd metacarpal
5, adductor pollicis muscle
6, dorsal interosseous muscle
7, palmar interosseous muscle

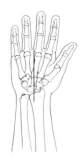

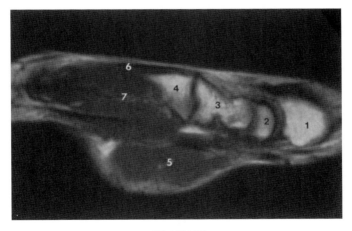

SE 2000/20

Extremity Coil
1, radius
2, lunate
3, capitate
4, 3rd metacarpal
5, flexor tendon
6, palmar interosseous muscle
7, pronator quadratus muscle

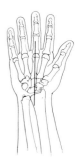

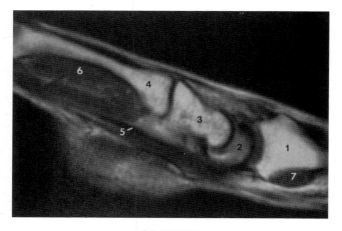

SE 2000/20

Body Coil

1, rectus abdominis muscle
2, anterior ilium
3, iliacus muscle
4, psoas muscle
5, multifidus and iliocostalis
   lumborum muscles
6, sacroiliac joint
7, sacrum
8, gluteus maximus muscle
9, gluteus medius muscle

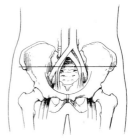

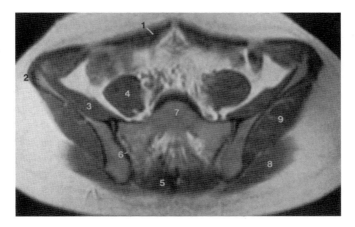

SE 500/20

Body Coil
1, rectus abdominis muscle
2, iliopsoas muscle
3, ilium
4, gluteus maximus muscle
5, gluteus medius muscle
6, gluteus minimus muscle
7, transverse abdominis
   muscle

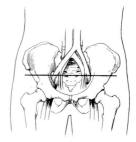

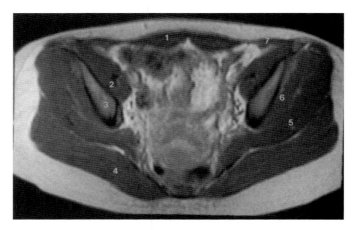

SE 500/20

Body Coil

1, rectus abdominis muscle
2, iliopsoas muscle
3, anterior inferior iliac spine
4, acetabulum
5, gluteus minimus muscle
6, gluteus maximus muscle
7, gluteus medius muscle
8, sartorius muscle
9, external iliac vessels

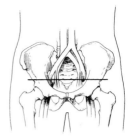

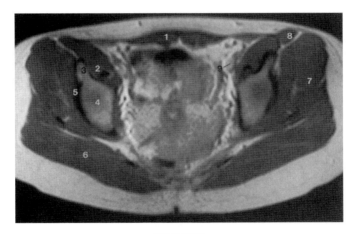

SE 500/20

Body Coil

1, femoral artery and vein
2, iliopsoas muscle
3, sartorius muscle
4, tensor fascia lata
5, rectus femoris muscle
6, gluteus maximus muscle
7, obturator internus muscle
8, ischium
9, sciatic nerve
10, gemellus inferior muscle
11, greater trochanter
12, femoral head
13, bladder

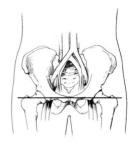

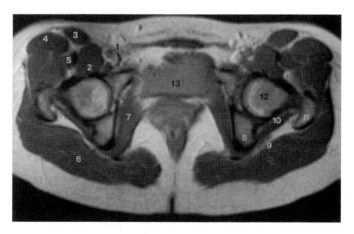

SE 500/20

Body Coil

1, pectineus muscle
2, femoral artery and vein
3, sartorius muscle
4, tensor fascia lata
5, rectus femoris muscle
6, femoral neck
7, gluteus maximus muscle
8, ischial tuberosity
9, obturator internus muscle
10, obturator externus muscle
11, vastus intermedius muscle
12, vastus lateralis muscle
13, sciatic nerve

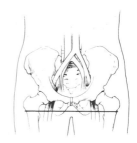

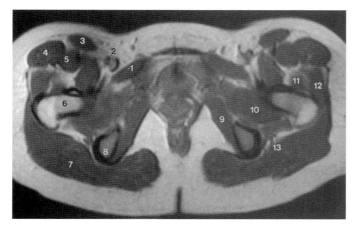

SE 500/20

Body Coil

1, pubic symphysis
2, iliacus muscle
3, tensor fascia lata
4, iliopsoas muscle
5, femoral artery and vein, and branch vessels
6, gluteus minimus muscle
7, gluteus medius muscle
8, pectineus muscle
9, adductor longus muscle
10, vastus intermedius muscle
11, vastus lateralis muscle

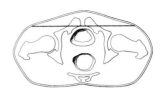

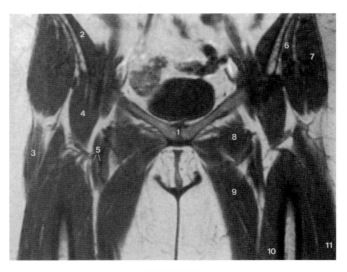

SE 500/20

Body Coil

1, iliacus muscle
2, gluteus minimus muscle
3, obturator internus muscle
4, obturator externus muscle
5, vastus lateralis muscle
6, greater trochanter
7, adductor muscle
8, gracilis muscle
9, bladder

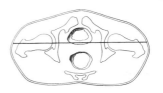

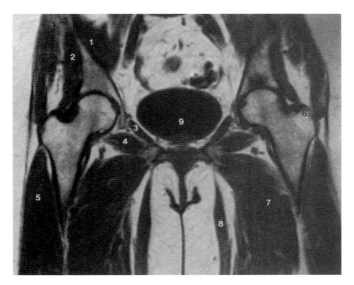

SE 500/20

Body Coil

1, sacroiliac joint
2, posterior acetabulum
3, quadratus femoris muscle
4, biceps femoris muscle
5, semitendinosus muscle
6, semimembranosis muscle
7, tensor facia lata
8, gluteus maximus muscle
9, rectum

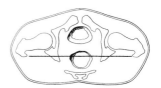

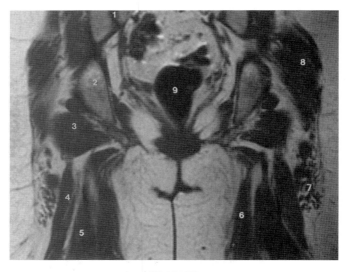

SE 500/20

Body Coil
1, rectus abdominis muscle
2, iliopsoas muscle
3, gluteus maximus muscle
4, ilium
5, ischial tuberosity
6, obturator externus muscle
7, rectus femoris muscle
8, superficial femoral artery
   and vein
9, ligamentum teres
10, adductor muscle
11, semimembranosis and
    semitendinosus muscles

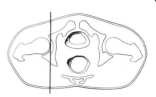

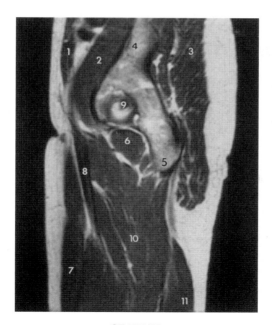

SE 500/20

Body Coil
1, iliopsoas muscle
2, acetabulum
3, femoral head
4, rectus femoris muscle
5, sartorius muscle
6, hamstring tendon origins
7, gluteus maximus muscle
8, semitendinosus muscle
9, adductor magnus muscle
10, obturator externus muscle
11, vastus intermedius muscle

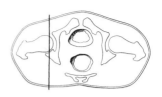

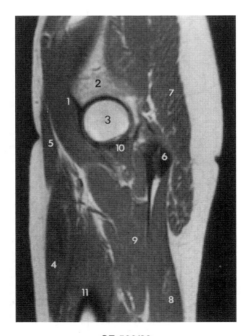

SE 500/20

Body Coil

1, femur
2, gluteus maximus muscle
3, gluteus medius muscle
4, gluteus minimus muscle
5, quadratus femoris muscle
6, rectus femoris muscle
7, vastus intermedius muscle
8, vastus lateralis muscle

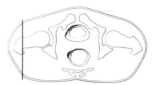

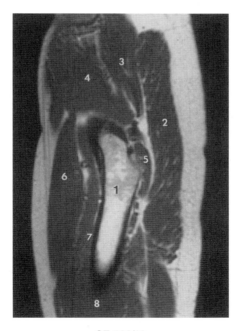

SE 500/20

Body Coil

1, saphenous veins
2, adductor longus muscle
3, gracilis muscle
4, adductor brevis muscle
5, adductor magnus muscle
6, semitendinosus muscle
7, gluteus maximus muscle
8, vastus lateralis muscle
9, vastus intermedius muscle
10, pectineus muscle
11, tensor fascia lata
12, rectus femoris
13, deep femoral artery and vein, and superficial femoral artery and vein
14, sartorius muscle

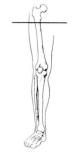

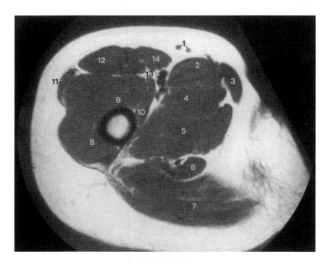

SE 500/20

Body Coil

1, sartorius muscle
2, superficial femoral artery and vein
3, saphenous veins
4, adductor longus muscle
5, gracilis muscle
6, deep femoral artery and vein
7, adductor brevis muscle
8, adductor magnus muscle
9, semitendinosus muscle
10, medial fascia
11, sciatic nerve
12, gluteus maximus muscle
13, biceps femoris muscle
14, vastus lateralis muscle
15, vastus intermedius and medialis muscles
16, rectus femoris muscle

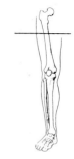

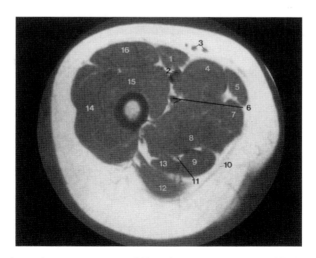

Lateral   SE 500/20   Medial

Body Coil
1, rectus femoris muscle
2, vastus medialis muscle
3, sartorius muscle
4, greater saphenous vein
5, superficial femoral artery
  and vein
6, adductor longus muscle
7, adductor magnus muscle
8, gracilis muscle
9, semimembranosus muscle
10, semitendinosus muscle
11, biceps femoris (long head)
12, sciatic nerve
13, biceps femoris (short head)
14, vastus lateralis muscle
15, vastus intermedius muscle

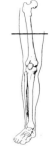

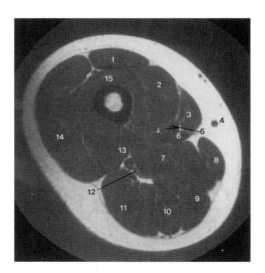

Lateral   SE 500/20   Medial

Body Coil
1, gluteus maximus muscle
2, ischial tuberosity
3, tendon for hamstring muscles
4, biceps femoris muscle
5, femoral artery
6, gracilis muscle
7, biceps femoris tendon

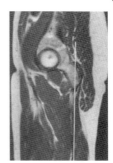

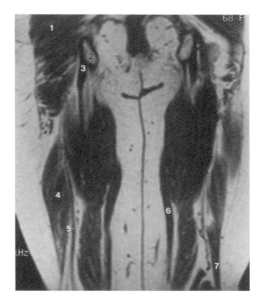

Right   SE 500/20   Left

Body Coil
1, right femur
2, left femur
3, iliotibial tract
4, iliotibial band
5, vastus intermedius muscle
6, gracilis muscle
7, obturator internus muscle
8, obturator externus muscle
9, adductor muscles

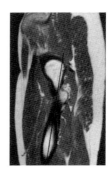

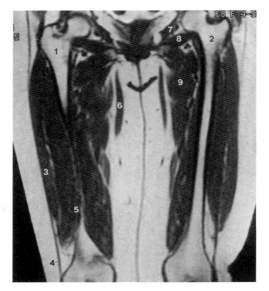

Right   SE 500/20   Left

Extremity Coil
1, quadriceps tendon
2, vastus medialis muscle
3, sartorius muscle
4, greater saphenous vein
5, gracilis muscle
6, semimembranosus muscle
7, semitendinosus muscle
8, popliteal artery and vein
9, tibial nerve
10, biceps femoris muscle
11, vastus lateralis muscle

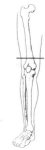

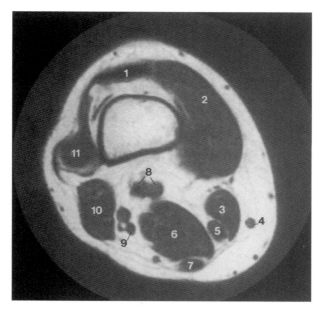

Lateral   SE 500/20   Medial

Extremity Coil

1, patella
2, medial retinaculum
3, medial collateral ligament
4, sartorius muscle
5, greater saphenous vein
6, gracilis tendon
7, semitendinosus muscle
8, semimembranosus muscle
9, gastrocnemius muscle (medial)
10, popliteal artery and vein
11, tibial nerve
12, gastrocnemius muscle (lateral)
13, biceps femoris muscle and tendon
14, lateral retinaculum

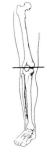

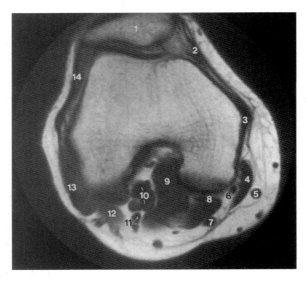

Lateral   SE 500/20   Medial

Extremity Coil

1, patellar tendon
2, medial collateral ligament
3, sartorius muscle and tendon
4, gracilis tendon
5, semimembranosus tendon
6, semitendinosus tendon
7, gastrocnemius muscle (medial)
8, popliteal artery
9, tibial nerve
10, gastrocnemius muscle (lateral)
11, common peroneal nerve
12, biceps femoris tendon
13, lateral collateral ligament
14, lateral meniscus

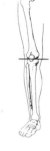

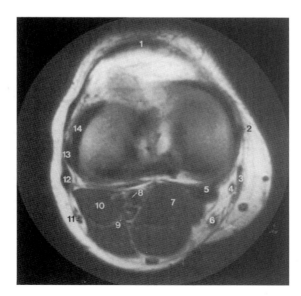

Lateral   SE 500/20   Medial

Extremity Coil
1, patellar tendon
2, tibia
3, greater saphenous vein
4, semitendinosus tendon
5, gastrocnemius muscle
   (medial)
6, small saphenous vein
7, gastrocnemius muscle
   (lateral)
8, biceps femoris tendon

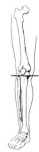

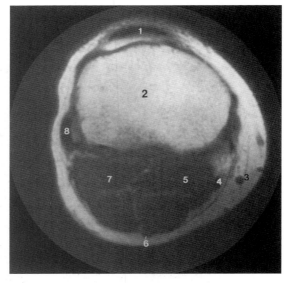

Lateral   SE 500/20   Medial

Extremity Coil

1, fibula
2, tibia
3, popliteus muscle
4, greater saphenous vein
5, gastrocnemius muscle
   (medial)
6, small saphenous vein
7, gastrocnemius muscle
   (lateral)
8, biceps femoris tendon

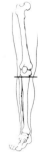

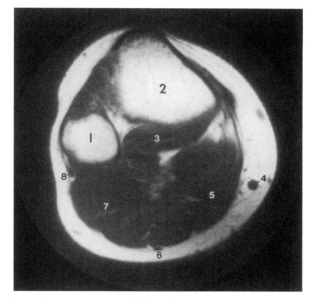

Lateral   SE 500/20   Medial

Extremity Coil

1, lateral gastrocnemius muscle
2, biceps femoris muscle
3, fibular head
4, soleus muscle
5, medial gastrocnemius muscle
6, medial femoral condyle
7, superior geniculate vessels
8, popliteal artery

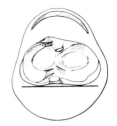

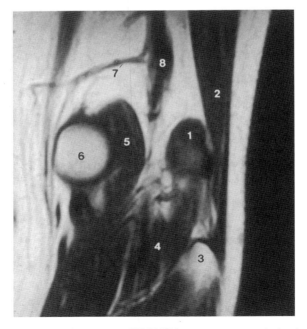

Medial   SE 500/20   Lateral

Extremity Coil
1, medial femoral condyle
2, medial head
gastrocnemius muscle
3, ligament of Wrisberg
4, lateral femoral condyle
5, biceps femoris muscle
6, biceps femoris tendon
7, fibular head
8, popliteus muscle
9, posterior cruciate ligament
10, semimembranosus tendon
11, gastrocnemius muscle
(medial)

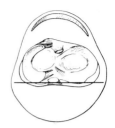

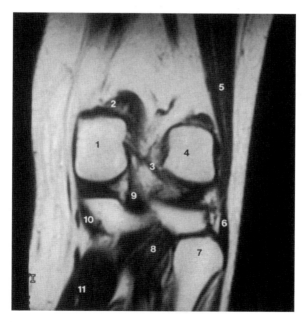

Medial   SE 500/20   Lateral

Extremity Coil

1, medial collateral ligament
2, medial femoral condyle
3, posterior cruciate ligament
4, anterior cruciate ligament
5, lateral meniscus
6, iliotibial tract
7, peroneus longus muscle

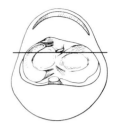

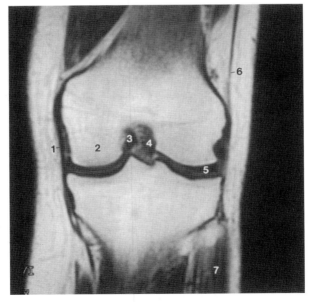

Medial   SE 500/20   Lateral

Extremity Coil
1, lateral femoral condyle
2, lateral head of
   gastrocnemius muscle
3, popliteal tendon
4, lateral meniscus
5, fibular head
6, soleus muscle
7, extensor digitorum longus
   muscle

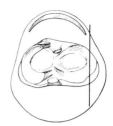

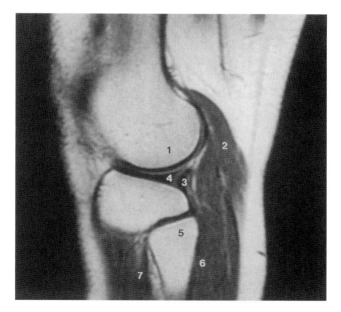

Medial   SE 500/20   Lateral

Extremity Coil
1, patellar tendon
2, patella
3, quadriceps tendon
4, gastrocnemius muscle
5, posterior cruciate ligament
6, anterior cruciate ligament
7, infrapatellar fat
8, popliteus muscle
9, soleus muscle

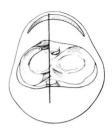

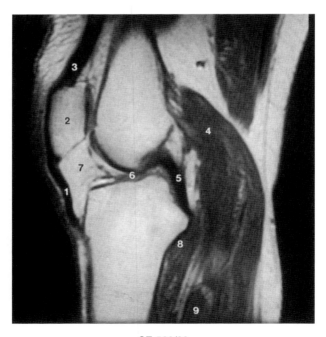

SE 500/20

Extremity Coil

1, medial femoral condyle
2, medial meniscus
3, semimembranosus tendon
4, semitendinosus tendon
5, medial gastrocnemius
6, vastus medialis muscle
7, semimembranosus muscle
8, semitendinosus muscle

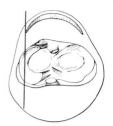

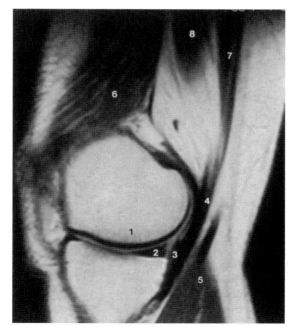

SE 500/20

Extremity Coil

1, tibia
2, fibula
3, flexor digitorum longus muscle
4, soleus muscle
5, medial gastrocnemius muscle
6, lateral gastrocnemius muscle
7, flexor hallucis longus muscle
8, posterior tibial artery, vein and nerve
9, peroneal artery and vein
10, tibialis posterior muscle
11, anterior tibial artery, vein and deep peroneal nerve
12, peroneus longus and brevis muscles

13, extensor digitorum longus muscle
14, tibialis anterior muscle

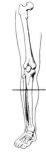

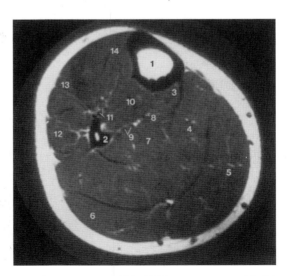

Lateral   SE 500/20   Medial

Extremity Coil

1, tibia
2, fibula
3, tibialis posterior muscle
4, flexor digitorum longus muscle
5, posterior tibial artery, vein and nerve
6, soleus muscle
7, medial gastrocnemius muscle
8, lesser saphenous vein
9, peroneus longus and brevis muscles
10, extensor digitorum longus muscle
11, tibialis anterior muscle

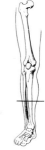

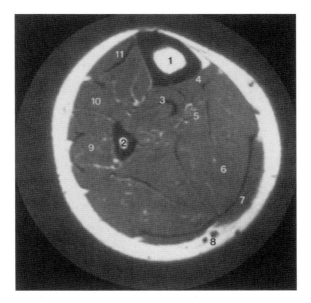

Lateral   SE 500/20   Medial

Extremity Coil

1, tibia
2, fibula
3, tibialis posterior muscle
4, flexor digitorum longus muscle
5, posterior tibial artery, vein and nerve
6, soleus muscle
7, gastrocnemius aponeurosis
8, peroneus longus and brevis muscles
9, flexor hallucis longus muscle
10, extensor digitorum longus muscle
11, extensor hallucis longus muscle
12, tibialis anterior muscle

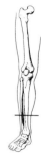

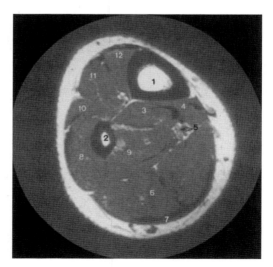

Lateral   Medial

Extremity Coil

1, tibia
2, fibula
3, tibialis posterior tendon
4, flexor digitorum longus muscle
5, posterior tibial artery, vein and nerve
6, Achilles tendon
7, sural nerve
8, peroneal muscles and tendons
9, extensor digitorum longus muscle
10, extensor hallucis longus muscle
11, tibialis anterior muscle

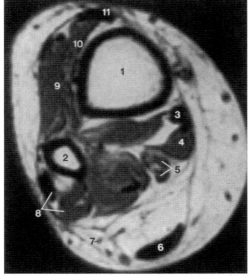

Lateral   SE 500/20   Medial

Extremity Coil

1, tibia
2, fibula
3, tibialis anterior tendon
4, tibialis posterior tendon
5, flexor digitorum longus tendon
6, flexor hallucis longus tendon
7, posterior tibial artery, vein and nerve
8, Achilles tendon
9, peroneus brevis and longus tendons
10, extensor hallucis longus tendon

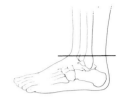

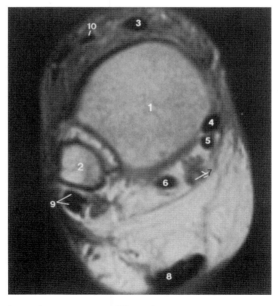

Lateral   SE 500/20   Medial

Extremity Coil

1, tibia
2, fibula
3, tibialis anterior tendon
4, tibialis posterior tendon
5, flexor digitorum longus tendon
6, hallucis longus tendon
7, posterior tibial artery, vein and nerve
8, Achilles tendon
9, peroneus brevis and longus tendons
10, extensor hallucis longus tendon
11, extensor digitorum longus tendons

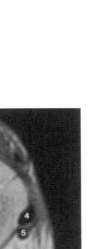

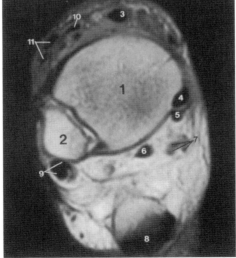

Lateral   SE 500/20   Medial

Extremity Coil

1, medial malleolus
2, lateral malleolus
3, tibialis anterior tendon
4, tibialis posterior tendon
5, flexor digitorum longus
   tendon
6, flexor hallucis longus
   tendon
7, calcaneus
8, posterior tibial artery, vein
   and nerve
9, peroneus brevis and longus
   tendons

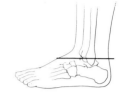

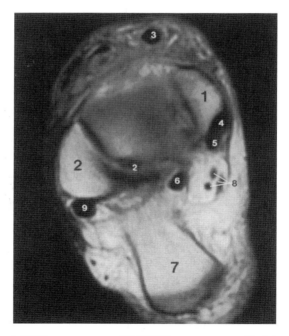

Lateral   SE 500/20   Medial

Extremity Coil
1, talus
2, calcaneus
3, tibialis anterior tendon
4, tibialis posterior tendon
5, flexor digitorum longus
   tendon
6, flexor hallucis longus
   tendon
7, peroneal tendons
8, extensor hallucis longus
   tendon
9, anterior tibial artery

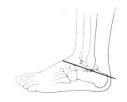

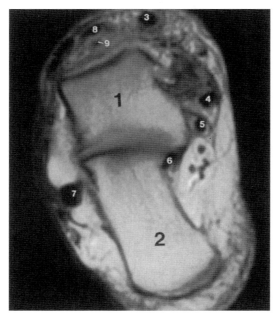

Lateral   SE 500/20   Medial

Extremity Coil
1, talus
2, calcaneus
3, sustentaculum tali
4, tibialis anterior tendon
5, tibialis posterior tendon
6, flexor digitorum longus tendon
7, flexor hallucis longus tendon
8, peroneus brevis tendon
9, peroneus longus tendon
10, extensor hallucis longus tendon
11, dorsalis pedis artery
12, extensor digitorum longus tendons

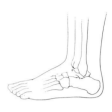

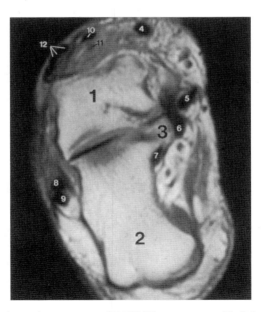

Lateral   SE 500/20   Medial

Extremity Coil

1, calcaneus
2, flexor hallucis longus
   muscle
3, peroneus brevis muscle
4, quadratus plantae muscle
5, abductor hallucis muscle
6, plantar aponeurosis
7, pre-Achilles fat pad

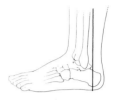

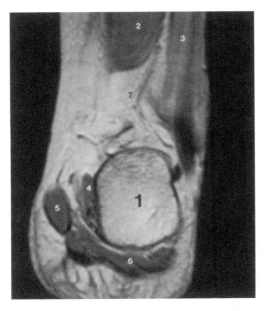

Medial   SE 2000/20   Lateral

Extremity Coil

1, fibula
2, tibia
3, calcaneus
4, tibialis posterior muscle
5, flexor digitorum longus tendon
6, abductor hallucis muscle
7, flexor digitorum brevis muscle
8, abductor digiti minimi muscle
9, peroneus longus tendon
10, peroneus brevis tendon
11, calcaneofibular ligament
12, posterior distal tibiofibular ligament

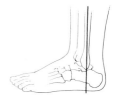

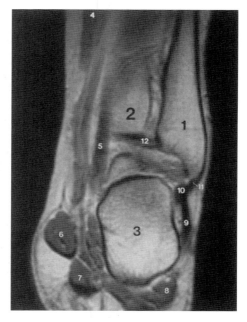

Medial   SE 2000/20   Lateral

Extremity Coil

1, tibia
2, talus
3, sustentaculum tali
4, calcaneus
5, tibiotalar ligament
6, tibiocalcaneal ligament
7, tibialis posterior tendon
8, flexor digitorum longus
   tendon
9, flexor hallucis longus
   tendon
10, abductor hallucis muscle

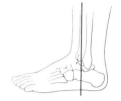

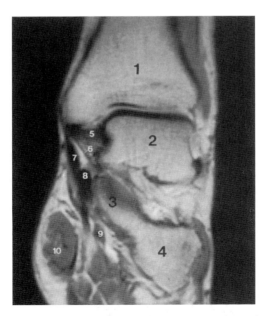

Medial   SE 2000/20   Lateral

Extremity Coil

1, navicular
2, cuboid
3, flexor hallucis brevis
   muscle
4, flexor hallucis longus
   tendon
5, flexor digitorum longus
   tendon
6, medial plantar artery, vein
   and nerve
7, abductor digiti minimi
   muscle
8, peroneus longus tendon
9, peroneus brevis tendon

10, extensor digitorum longus
    tendons
11, extensor hallucis longus
    tendons
12, tibialis anterior tendon

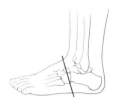

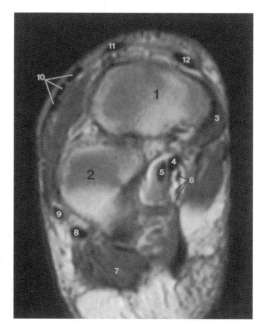

Lateral   SE 2000/20   Medial

Extremity Coil

1, cuboid
2, lateral cuneiform
3, intermediate cuneiform
4, medial cuneiform
5, peroneus brevis tendon
6, peroneus longus tendon
7, abductor digiti minimi muscle
8, lateral plantar artery, vein and nerve
9, flexor digitorum brevis muscle
10, flexor hallucis and flexor digitorum longus tendons
11, abductor hallucis muscle
12, tibialis anterior tendon
13, extensor hallucis longus tendon
14, extensor digitorum longus tendons

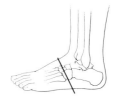

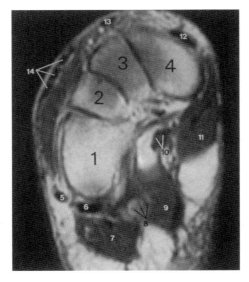

Lateral   SE 2000/20   Medial

Extremity Coil

1–5, 1st through 5th metatarsals
   6, extensor hallucis longus tendon
   7, abductor hallucis muscle
   8, flexor hallucis brevis muscle
   9, adductor hallucis muscle
  10, flexor digitorum brevis muscle
  11, flexor digitorum longus tendons
  12, flexor digiti minimi brevis muscle
  13, abductor digiti minimi muscle

14, dorsal interosseus muscle 2
15, dorsal interosseus muscle 4

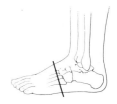

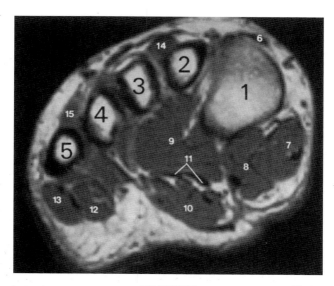

Lateral   SE 2000/20   Medial

Extremity Coil

1–5, 1st through 5th metatarsals
6, extensor hallucis longus tendon
7, abductor hallucis muscle
8, flexor hallucis brevis muscle
9, flexor hallucis longus tendon
10, adductor hallucis muscle
11, flexor digitorum brevis muscle
12, plantar interosseous muscles
13, flexor digiti minimi brevis muscle

14, abductor digiti minimi muscle

di, dorsal interosseous muscles

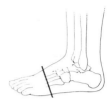

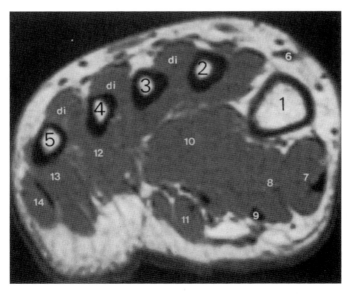

Lateral   SE 2000/20   Medial

Extremity Coil
1, tibia
2, talus
3, sustentaculum tali
4, calcaneus
5, navicular
6, medial cuneiform
7, artery of the tarsal canal
8, flexor hallucis longus tendon
9, abductor hallucis muscle
10, Achilles tendon

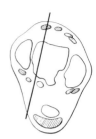

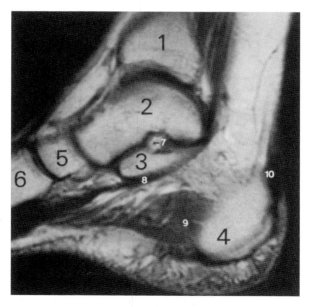

SE 500/20

Extremity Coil

1, tibia
2, talus
3, navicular
4, calcaneus
5, flexor hallucis longus muscle
6, soleus muscle
7, Achilles tendon
8, talocalcaneal interosseous ligament
9, quadratus plantae muscle
10, flexor digitorum brevis muscle

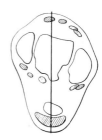

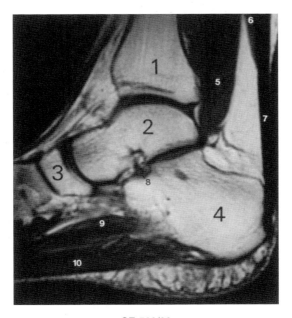

SE 500/20

Extremity Coil
1, fibula
2, peroneus brevis tendon
3, peroneus longus tendon

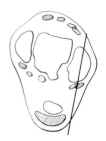

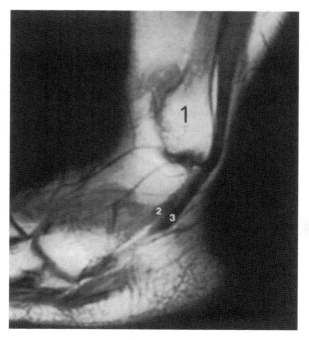

SE 500/20

Extremity Coil

1, 1st metatarsal
2, medial cuneiform
3, navicular
4, sustentaculum tali
5, abductor hallucis muscle
6, flexor hallucis brevis muscle
7, flexor hallucis longus
   tendon

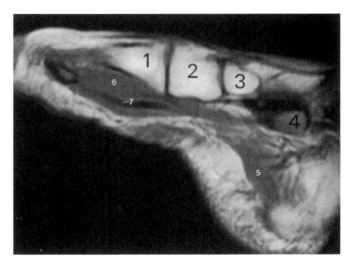

SE 500/20

Extremity Coil
1, 2nd metatarsal
2, intermediate cuneiform
3, navicular
4, talus
5, calcaneus
6, flexor digitorum brevis muscle
7, flexor digitorum longus tendon
8, adductor hallucis muscle

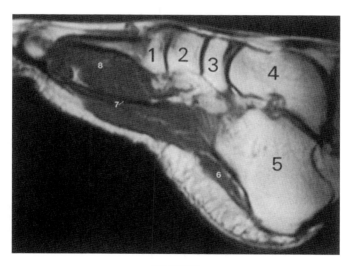

SE 500/20

Extremity Coil
1, lateral cuneiform
2, cuboid
3, talus
4, calcaneus
5, tarsal canal
6, abductor digiti minimi
   muscle
7, plantar interosseous muscle

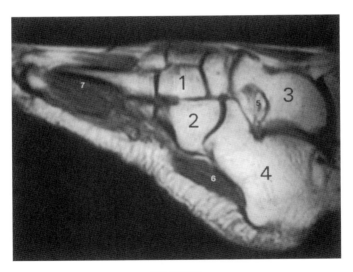

SE 500/20

Extremity Coil

1, peroneus brevis tendon
2, peroneus longus tendon
3, 5th metatarsal
4, dorsal interosseous muscle
5, flexor digiti minimi brevis
   muscle

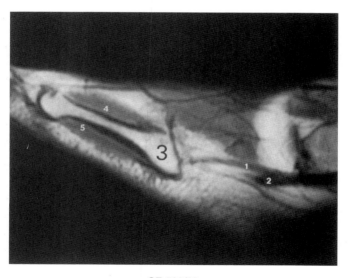

SE 500/20

Bibliography

1. Beltran J, Noto AM, Mosure JC, Weiss KL, Zuelzcr W, Christoforidis AJ: The knee: surface coil MR imaging at 1.5 T. *Radiology* 1986;159:747–751.
2. Cahill DR, Orland MJ: *Atlas of Luman Cross-Sectional Anatomy.* 1984; Philadelphia, Lea & Febiger.
3. Erickson SJ, Rosengarten JL: MR imaging of the forefoot: normal anatomic findings. *AJR* 1993;160:565–571.
4. Grant JCB: *Grant's Atlas of Anatomy.* 1962; Baltimore, Williams & Wilkins.
5. Holliday J, Saxon R, Lufken RB, Rauschning CV, Reicher M, Bassett L, Hanafel W, Barbarie Z, Santi D, Glenn W: Anatomic correlations of magnetic resonance images with cadaver cryosections. *Radiographics* 1985; 5:887–921.
6. Kang HS, Resnick D: *MRI of the Extremities: An Anatomic Atlas.* 1991; Philadelphia, WB Saunders Co.
7. Kieft GJ, Bloein JL, Obermann WR, Verbout AJ, Rozurg PM, Doornvas J: Normal shoulder: MR imaging. *Radiology* 1986;159:741–745.
8. Link SC, Erickson SJ, Tumins ME: MR imaging of the ankle and foot: normal structure and anatomic variants that may simulate disease. *AJR* 1993;161:607–612.